ESSENTIAL 101 TIPS

YOGA

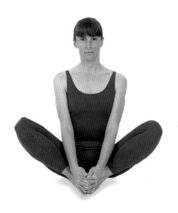

D1115467

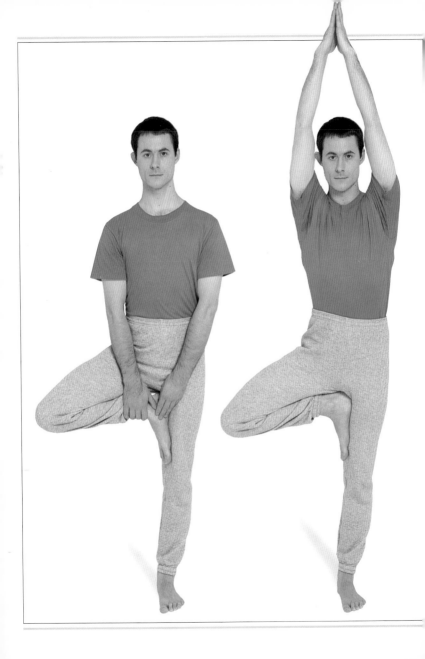

ESSENTIAL TIPS

YOGA

Sivananda Yoga Vedanta Centre

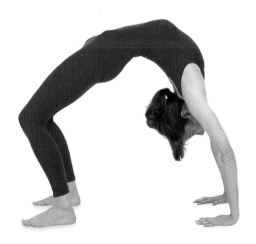

LONDON, NEW YORK, MELBOURNE,
MUNICH AND DELHI

Editor Lucinda Hawksley, Ian Whitelaw
Art Editor Elaine Hewson
Managing Editor Gillian Roberts
Managing Art Editor Karen Sawyer
Category Publisher Mary-Clare Jerram
DTP Designer Sonia Charbonnier
Production Controller Luca Frassinetti

First American edition, 1995
This paperback edition published in the United States in 2003
by DK Publishing, Inc.
375 Hudson Street, New York, New York 10014
Penguin Group (US)

A Cataloging-in-Publication record for this book is available from the Library of Congress

ISBN 0–7894–9684–4

Color reproduced in Singapore by Colourscan
Printed in Hong Kong by Wing King Tong

See our complete product line at
www.dk.com

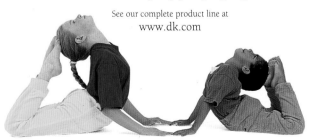

ESSENTIAL TIPS
101

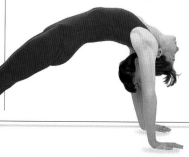

PREPARATION

1 WHAT IS YOGA?

The word *yoga* means "union." Yoga is a form of exercise based on the belief that the body and breath are intimately connected with the mind. By controlling the breath and holding the body in steady poses, or *asanas*, yoga creates harmony.

Yoga practice consists of five key elements: proper breathing, proper exercise, proper relaxation, proper diet, and positive thinking and meditation. The exercises, or asanas, are designed to ease tensed muscles, to tone up the internal organs, and to improve the flexibility of the body's joints and ligaments.

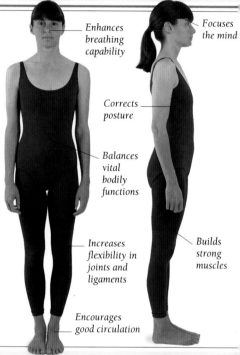

Enhances breathing capability

Focuses the mind

Corrects posture

Balances vital bodily functions

Increases flexibility in joints and ligaments

Builds strong muscles

Encourages good circulation

2 CHECK WITH YOUR DOCTOR

Yoga asanas can be practiced by young and old alike. While there is no one who should be excluded, check with your doctor before you begin a course if you suffer from a medical condition or have any doubts.

3 PROPER EXERCISE: YOGA ASANAS

The aim of proper exercise is to improve suppleness and strength. Each posture is performed slowly in fluid movements. Violent movements are avoided; they produce a buildup of lactic acid, causing fatigue.

4 PROPER BREATHING

Most people use only a fraction of their breathing capacity. Proper breathing focuses on nasal breathing techniques to unlock energy and vitality. Breathing exercises concentrate on exhalation rather than inhalation, to cleanse the lungs of stale air and to eliminate toxins from the body.

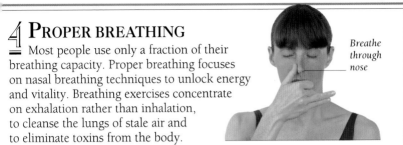

Breathe through nose

5 PROPER RELAXATION

The release of tension through relaxation is vital to keep the body healthy. Begin and end each session of yoga asanas with relaxation, and relax between postures. This allows the released energy to flow freely.

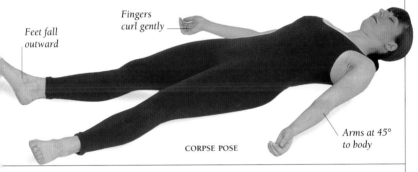

Fingers curl gently

Feet fall outward

CORPSE POSE

Arms at 45° to body

6 PROPER DIET

The recommended diet for a student of yoga is a simple and wholesome vegetarian one, made up of natural foods that are easily digested. It keeps the body vital and healthy, and the mind calm and free from restless thoughts. Processed and canned foods are to be avoided when possible.

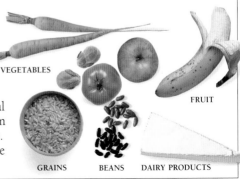

VEGETABLES

FRUIT

GRAINS   BEANS   DAIRY PRODUCTS

9

7 POSITIVE THINKING & MEDITATION

Meditation is a state of consciousness. When practicing meditation, you must first learn how to calm the mind and focus your mental energy inward. Meditation can help relieve stress and replenish your energy. If it is practiced on a daily basis, you will also find that it will enable you to think more clearly and positively, and to be at peace with yourself.

Focus the mind

Rest hands on knees

SITTING POSITION ▷
An advanced yoga student will sit in the Lotus Position (see p.36) when meditating. If you are a beginner, you will find it much easier to sit in the Comfortable Cross-legged Position (see p.59).

8 THE IMPORTANCE OF A TEACHER

Whether you are learning yoga singly or in a group, it is always best to be supervised by a qualified teacher. A teacher will demonstrate how to ease your body gently into and out of the yoga postures and, most importantly, how to breathe correctly when holding a balance. He or she will ensure that you do not strain your limbs and will help you align your body in the asanas.

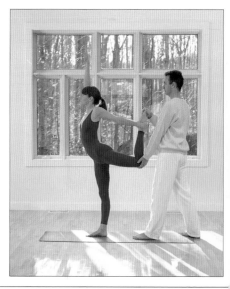

PROPER SUPERVISION ▷
As well as helping you correct and improve your technique, an expert will help you build confidence in your ability to perform asanas.

9 WHAT YOU NEED

You do not need special equipment to practice yoga. Although you can buy special yoga mats, a towel on a carpeted floor will do just as well. For practicing indoors, you will need an open space without furniture. The room should be comfortably heated and free from disturbances.

READY TO BEGIN
Remove jewelry, glasses, and contact lenses, if practical, before starting a yoga session.

△ **EXTRA EQUIPMENT**
Practice on a rug or towel for comfort. A blanket and heater will keep you warm during relaxation periods.

△ **WHAT TO WEAR**
Clothing should be comfortable so that you have total freedom of movement. It is best to practice yoga in bare feet, but if you suffer from the cold, you can wear socks.

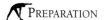
10 WHEN & WHERE TO PRACTICE

Try to practice yoga every day. At the same time, be gentle. Do not force yourself. A yoga session should be a joy. Set aside a time when you will not be disturbed and you will not have to rush. Practicing in the morning helps loosen stiff joints after sleep. Practicing in the evening relieves the tensions of the day. Whenever you practice yoga, avoid eating for at least two hours beforehand.

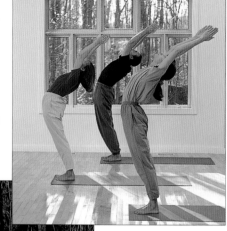

△ INDOOR PRACTICE
If practicing inside, choose a peaceful, spacious location. Yoga classes offer mutual encouragement and help develop group energy.

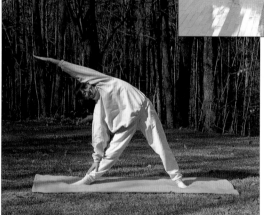

◁ OUTDOOR PRACTICE
Yoga balances the mind and body, so try to choose a complementary location. A beautiful, natural setting that calms the mind is the perfect place to practice.

11 EACH SESSION: HOW LONG?

For maximum benefit, you should set aside about 90 minutes. When you are busy, try a shorter session with fewer asanas. It is very important not to feel rushed and to allow time for relaxation between poses. You can always perform the breathing exercises at a later stage.

12 KNOW YOUR BODY'S CAPABILITIES

Before you begin your yoga asanas, it is important to recognize your body's capabilities. Never force your body into a posture or try to go beyond your limit. Remember, yoga is not a competitive sport. Progress may be slow, but with time your body will become flexible. Ease yourself gently into each position, and when you are holding a pose, check the body to see if you can feel tension building up anywhere. If you do, consciously try to relax that tension using the breathing.

13 BALANCING BOTH SIDES OF THE BODY

Many of our regular daily activities tend to emphasize the use of one part or side of the body. To achieve a healthy and harmonious balance, it is important to keep all parts of the body equally strong and flexible. Yoga exercises make each group of muscles work equally on the left and right sides of the body to achieve equilibrium.

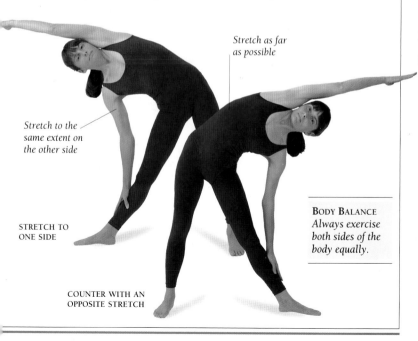

Stretch as far as possible

Stretch to the same extent on the other side

STRETCH TO ONE SIDE

BODY BALANCE
Always exercise both sides of the body equally.

COUNTER WITH AN OPPOSITE STRETCH

BREATHING TECHNIQUES

14 THE IMPORTANCE OF PROPER BREATHING

Breathing gives life. Without oxygen no human cell can live for more than a few minutes. Many people use only part of their full breathing capacity, taking in about one third of the oxygen that their lungs could use. This leads to stress and fatigue. The yogic breath discipline teaches you to breathe through the nose, to accentuate exhalation rather than inhalation, to cleanse the lungs and eliminate toxins. These techniques increase your physical and mental health.

15 HOW THE LUNGS WORK

On an inhalation, your diaphragm (situated below the lungs) moves downward. Air you breathe in through the nose is drawn down the trachea to the lungs, which are protected by the rib cage. If you are breathing properly, the abdomen and rib cage will expand as you inhale. On an exhalation, your diaphragm moves upward, compressing the lungs and pushing air out of them. The air passes back up through the trachea and out through the nostrils.

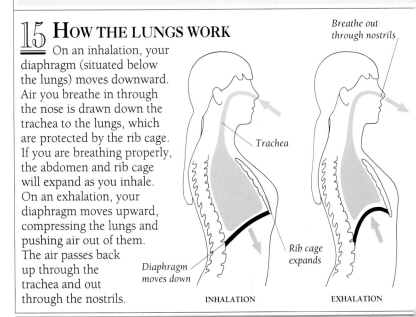

Breathe out through nostrils

Trachea

Rib cage expands

Diaphragm moves down

INHALATION

EXHALATION

16 ABDOMINAL BREATHING

Learn to breathe efficiently. Lie flat on your back, placing one hand on your abdomen. Start to inhale deeply, feeling your abdomen rise; then feel it fall as you exhale. Breathing slowly and deeply brings air to the lowest part of your lungs and exercises your diaphragm.

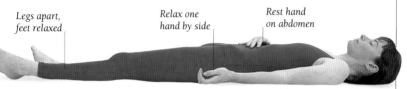

Legs apart, feet relaxed

Relax one hand by side

Rest hand on abdomen

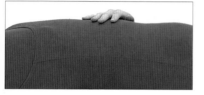

BREATHE IN

BREATHE OUT

17 SITTING PROPERLY

Adopt this posture for the breathing exercises in Tips 18 to 21. Sit cross-legged, aligning your head, neck, and spine. Keep your shoulders straight but relaxed. If you are a beginner, sit on a cushion. This lifts the hips and makes it easier to keep the back straight.

Legs crossed comfortably

18 FULL YOGIC BREATH

Place one hand on your lower rib cage and one on your abdomen. Breathe in, trying to fill the lowest part of your lungs, then the middle, and then the top. Feel your chest and abdomen expand.

With hand on abdomen, feel it expand and contract

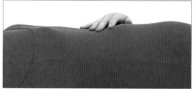

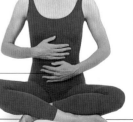

15

19 SINGLE NOSTRIL BREATHING

The object of practicing yogic breath discipline, or *Pranayama*, is to increase physical and mental health. You can practice the breathing exercises on their own or integrate them into your program of yoga asanas. Sit comfortably in a cross-legged position, with your spine and neck straight, but not tense.

Hold your head erect and gently close your eyes. Use the fingers of the right hand to close off each nostril in turn. Hold them in a position called Vishnu Mudra. For Vishnu Mudra, extend the thumb, ring finger, and little finger of your right hand and fold down your other two fingers into your palm. Rest the left hand on your left knee.

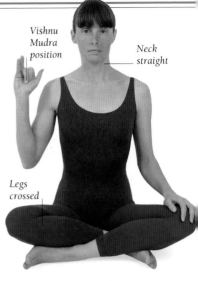

Vishnu Mudra position

Neck straight

Legs crossed

SIT AND BREATHE
This exercise is performed by breathing through one nostril at a time. The exhalation is longer than the inhalation.

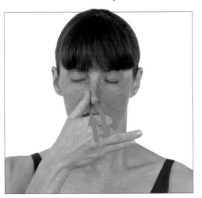

BREATHE THROUGH THE LEFT NOSTRIL
Close right nostril with thumb and inhale through left nostril to a count of four. Exhale to a count of eight. Repeat 10 times.

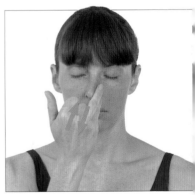

BREATHE THROUGH THE RIGHT NOSTRIL
Close left nostril with the two end fingers. Inhale through right nostril to a count of four and exhale to eight. Repeat 10 times.

20 ALTERNATE NOSTRIL BREATHING

When you are comfortable with Single Nostril Breathing, begin Alternate Nostril Breathing, where you practice retaining the breath for a count of 16. The action of Alternate Nostril Breathing is physical, but the greatest benefit is the calmness and lucidity of mind that results. Try to perform at least 10 rounds daily for best results.

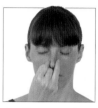

1 Inhale through the left nostril to a count of four.

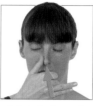

2 Close nostrils and hold breath to a count of 16.

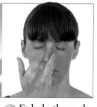

3 Exhale through the right nostril to a count of eight.

4 Inhale through the right nostril to a count of four.

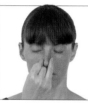

5 Close nostrils and hold breath to a count of 16.

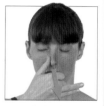

6 Exhale through the left nostril to a count of eight.

21 KAPALABHATI

This exercise, using rapid breathing, is believed to be such a powerful cleanser that the face literally "glows" with good health. Before beginning the exercise, relax by taking a few deep breaths. Perform 25 rapid "pumpings" in each round. Relax between rounds by breathing deeply. Try to do three rounds.

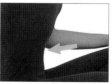

1 △ Force the air out of your lungs by rapidly contracting the muscles of your abdomen.

2 ▷ Relax the abdomen, allowing the lungs to fill with air. Do not force the inhalation.

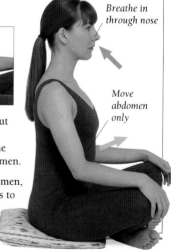

Breathe in through nose

Move abdomen only

STARTING-UP EXERCISES

22 EYE EXERCISES

Exercising the eyes releases any buildup of tension and aids relaxation. When practicing, keep your head still and move only your eyes.

MOVE EYES ▷
With eyes wide, look from side to side 10 times, then up and down 10 times, and then diagonally 10 times.

LOOK AHEAD ▷
Stare at your thumb, then look into the distance. Relax and repeat.

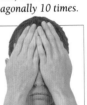

◁ COVER UP
Finally, after rolling your eyes in circles in both directions, cup your hands over your eyes for 30 seconds and relax.

23 NECK EXERCISES

Relax your neck muscles by combining these four exercises.

Sit cross-legged and practice each set of neck exercises at least three times.

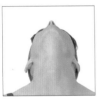
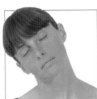

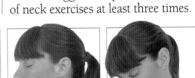

BACK AND FORTH
Drop your head back gently and then slowly drop it forward.

SIDE TO SIDE
Tilt your head to the right shoulder, to the center, and to the left.

TURN YOUR HEAD
Turn your head to look over each shoulder in turn.

CIRCLING
Inhale as you rotate your head to one side exhale to the other.

24 PURPOSE OF THE SUN SALUTATION

The Sun Salutation is a 12-part warm-up exercise. It limbers up the body and mind in preparation for the ensuing yoga session. Each of the 12 positions brings a different vertebral movement to the spinal column and is tuned to the inhalation or exhalation of the breath, thereby instilling a feeling of balance and harmony. The positions follow one after the other, making this Salutation graceful to perform. Attempt to do at least six sequences at the start of every session.

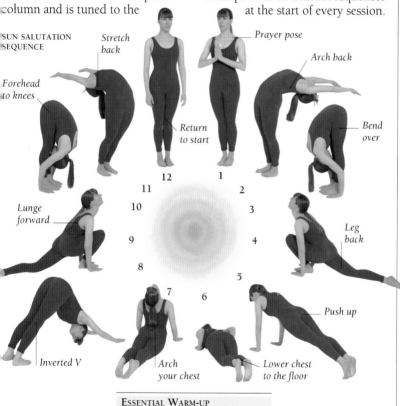

SUN SALUTATION SEQUENCE

Stretch back

Prayer pose

Arch back

Forehead to knees

Return to start

Bend over

Lunge forward

Leg back

Push up

Inverted V

Arch your chest

Lower chest to the floor

1 2 3 4 5 6 7 8 9 10 11 12

ESSENTIAL WARM-UP
Practice the Sun Salutation at the start of every yoga session. Tune the sequence to your breath.

25 PRAYER POSE

Stand up straight with your feet together and your arms by your sides. Take a deep breath, and then exhale while bringing your palms together at chest level.

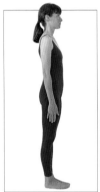

Feet together

STARTING POSITION

26 ARCH BACK

Inhale and stretch your arms up over your head. Arch your back so your hips come forward, and stretch as far as is comfortable.

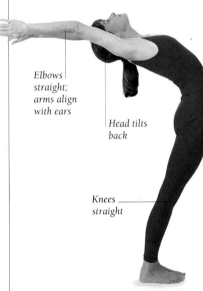

Elbows straight; arms align with ears

Head tilts back

Knees straight

27 BEND OVER

Exhale as you stretch forward and bend down into the third Sun Salutation position. Bring your hands down to the floor, and place them next to your feet, with the palms downward. Your hips should be kept as high as possible. If necessary, bend your knees so you can touch the ground. Tuck your forehead in toward your knees.

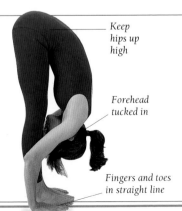

Keep hips up high

Forehead tucked in

Fingers and toes in straight line

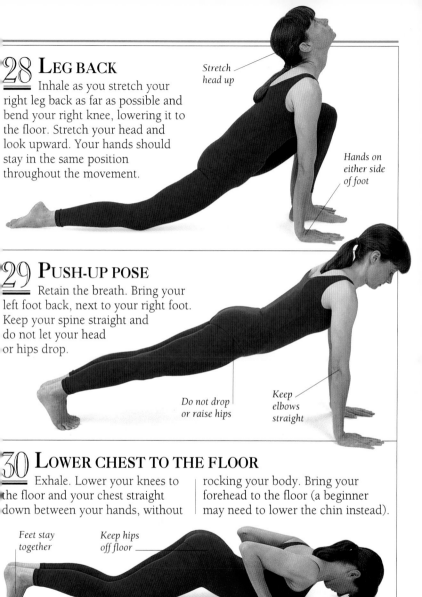

28 LEG BACK

Inhale as you stretch your right leg back as far as possible and bend your right knee, lowering it to the floor. Stretch your head and look upward. Your hands should stay in the same position throughout the movement.

Stretch head up

Hands on either side of foot

29 PUSH-UP POSE

Retain the breath. Bring your left foot back, next to your right foot. Keep your spine straight and do not let your head or hips drop.

Do not drop or raise hips

Keep elbows straight

30 LOWER CHEST TO THE FLOOR

Exhale. Lower your knees to the floor and your chest straight down between your hands, without rocking your body. Bring your forehead to the floor (a beginner may need to lower the chin instead).

Feet stay together

Keep hips off floor

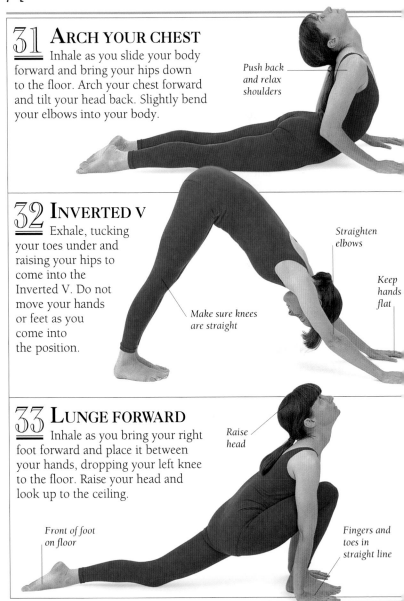

31 ARCH YOUR CHEST

Inhale as you slide your body forward and bring your hips down to the floor. Arch your chest forward and tilt your head back. Slightly bend your elbows into your body.

Push back and relax shoulders

32 INVERTED V

Exhale, tucking your toes under and raising your hips to come into the Inverted V. Do not move your hands or feet as you come into the position.

Straighten elbows

Keep hands flat

Make sure knees are straight

33 LUNGE FORWARD

Inhale as you bring your right foot forward and place it between your hands, dropping your left knee to the floor. Raise your head and look up to the ceiling.

Raise head

Front of foot on floor

Fingers and toes in straight line

34 FOREHEAD TO KNEES

Exhale as you bring your left foot forward and place it next to your right foot, so that the tips of your fingers and toes form a straight line. Raise your hips and stretch them upward, keeping your hands in the same position. If you cannot straighten your legs fully, allow your knees to remain slightly bent, but keep your hips up throughout. Bring your head down as far as possible and tuck it in as close to your knees as you can manage.

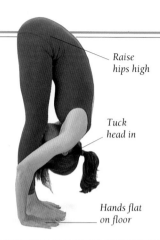

Raise hips high

Tuck head in

Hands flat on floor

35 STRETCH BACK

Inhale and then stand up, stretching your arms over your head as you straighten your body. Stretch your arms back, arch your chest and hips, and keep your feet together.

Hold arms parallel to ears

Arch chest forward

FULL STRETCH
Stretching the arms up above your head, arch your back into as full a curve as you can manage.

Keep knees straight

Feet together

36 RETURN TO START

Exhale and straighten up, lowering your arms to your sides. Now take a deep breath and prepare to begin another Sun Salutation sequence.

Hold body straight, but relaxed

BEGIN AGAIN
Starting the sequence again from Tip 25, this time lead with the left leg in Tips 28 and 33 (see pp.21 and 22).

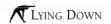
LYING DOWN

37 WHY DO THE CORPSE POSE?

The Corpse Pose is used at the beginning of a session to prepare you mentally and physically for the work ahead. It is also performed between postures to allow released energy to flow freely and to expel waste products from the muscles. Hold the pose for five minutes at the start and end of the session, and for a few minutes between poses.

38 HOW TO DO IT PROPERLY

Lie on your back with your heels at least 20 in (50 cm) apart and your toes falling outward. Your arms should be at approximately 45° to your body, with the palms of your hands facing upward. Close your eyes gently and lie still. Cover yourself with a blanket if you like.

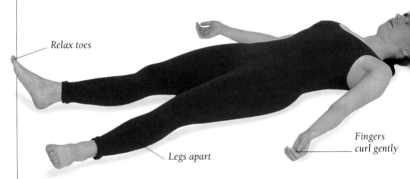

Relax toes

Legs apart

Fingers curl gently

39 THE PURPOSE OF LEG LIFTS

Leg Lifts strengthen your abdominal and lumbar muscles. By developing your physical strength it becomes easier to perform asanas correctly. When practicing Leg Lifts, keep your back pressed into the floor and relax your neck and shoulders. Keep your raised legs straight; lift them only to the point where you still feel comfortable.

40 SINGLE LEG LIFT

Start by lifting each leg three times. Synchronize each movement with the breath. Increase the lifts as the body becomes stronger.

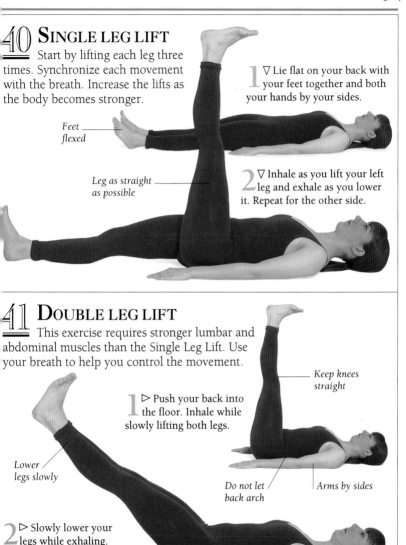

Feet flexed

Leg as straight as possible

1 ▽ Lie flat on your back with your feet together and both your hands by your sides.

2 ▽ Inhale as you lift your left leg and exhale as you lower it. Repeat for the other side.

41 DOUBLE LEG LIFT

This exercise requires stronger lumbar and abdominal muscles than the Single Leg Lift. Use your breath to help you control the movement.

Keep knees straight

1 ▷ Push your back into the floor. Inhale while slowly lifting both legs.

Lower legs slowly

Do not let back arch

Arms by sides

2 ▷ Slowly lower your legs while exhaling. Keep your legs as straight as possible. Start with five lifts and build up to 10.

25

HEADSTAND SEQUENCE

42 PURPOSE OF THE HEADSTAND

By inverting the entire body in the Headstand and balancing on your elbows, arms, and head, a plentiful supply of oxygen-rich blood can reach the upper regions of the body. The Headstand rests the heart, which usually has to work against gravity. This posture is referred to as the King of Asanas because of its many benefits for the body. It is considered by some to be a panacea for most human ills.

43 WHO SHOULD NOT DO A HEADSTAND

If you suffer from high blood pressure or have glaucoma, or any similar problems, do not attempt the Headstand. If you are not familiar with the Headstand, do not attempt it for the first time during pregnancy. If you are used to doing it, however, you can continue to practice this posture up until the fourth month, with your doctor's approval.

44 CHILD'S POSE

The Child's Pose is a simple relaxation posture that both comforts and relaxes your body in preparation for the Headstand (see p.28). Sit on your heels. Rest your forehead on the ground, and place your hands by your sides with the palms up. Breathe gently and relax.

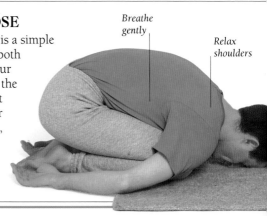

Breathe gently

Relax shoulders

15 DOLPHIN

The Dolphin strengthens the arms and shoulders in preparation for the Headstand. Start by sitting on your heels. Carefully position your forearms and straighten your legs. Push your body forward so that the chin comes in front of the hands, and then push back.

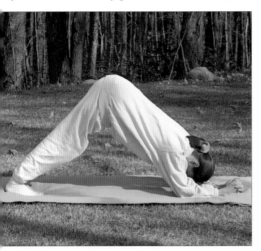

1 Sit on your heels with your toes pointing forward, and clasp each elbow with the opposite hand. Bring the elbows to the ground beneath the shoulders. Release the elbows and clasp your hands together in front of you. Now straighten your knees, raising the hips up.

2 Keeping your head off the ground, bring the chin as far in front of your hands as possible, and then push the body back. Repeat this 10 times.

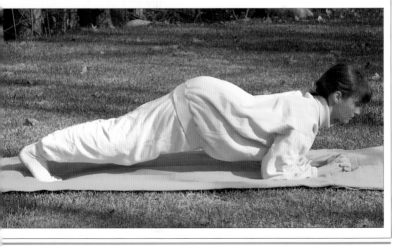

46 HEADSTAND

If you're not feeling confident enough to tackle the full Headstand, keep practicing the preliminary steps (1 to 6) to help prepare your body for the full posture. When you are able to balance for at least 30 secor with your knees tucked into your chest, you are ready to proceed.

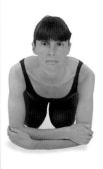

Legs and feet together

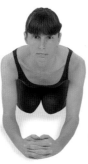

1 From the Child's Pose (*see p.26*), sit up on your heels and hold on to each elbow with your opposite hand.

2 Place your elbows on the floor below your shoulders and clasp your hands.

3 Position your arms to form a strong tripod. Lower your head so that the top of your skull touches the ground, and cradle the back of your head in your hands.

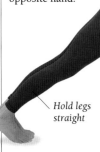

Hold legs straight

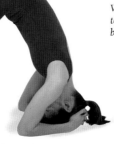

Walk feet toward body

4 Pushing your weight forward onto your forearms and elbows, rather than onto your head, straighten your knees and lift your bottom and hips up until you are standing on your toes.

5 When you are ready, slowly wa your feet in toward your head until your back is straight and you hips are directly over your head. D not bend your knees or drop the h

47 COMING OUT OF A HEADSTAND

In order to come out of the Headstand as carefully as you entered it, you should not exhaust yourself by holding the pose for too long. When you are ready to come down from the Headstand position, slowly bend your knees and gently lower them until your thighs are parallel with your chest. Straighten out your legs and lower your feet, your knees, and your body to the floor. You will end up back in the Child's Pose (see p.26). Rest like this for at least one minute.

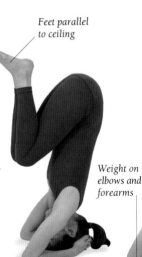

Feet parallel to ceiling

Weight on elbows and forearms

Legs held straight upward

Arch back slightly but tighten the abdominal muscles

6 Bend your knees and bring them into your chest. This is the Half-Headstand. Hold for 30 seconds before proceeding.

7 Keeping your knees bent, squeeze your stomach muscles to lift the hips gently until your knees point to the ceiling.

8 Straighten your knees and bring your feet up toward the ceiling. Breathe deeply and try to hold the Headstand for 30 seconds.

SHOULDERSTAND CYCLE

48 PURPOSE OF THE SHOULDERSTAND CYCLE

The Shoulderstand cycle strengthens the muscles, improves spinal flexibility, and balances the thyroid gland. This gland, in the neck, gives energy, equalizes the metabolism, controls body weight, removes poisons from the blood, and produces a radiant complexion

49 SHOULDERSTAND

This posture stretches your upper back muscles. Before starting, reach over your head to ensure that you have plenty of room behind you.

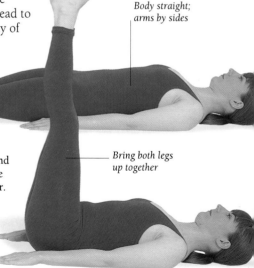

Body straight; arms by sides

Feet together

Bring both legs up together

1 △ Lie on your back with your arms by your sides and your palms facing down. Make sure that your feet are together.

2 ▷ Keeping your back on the ground, inhale as you raise your legs to an angle of 90° from the floor.

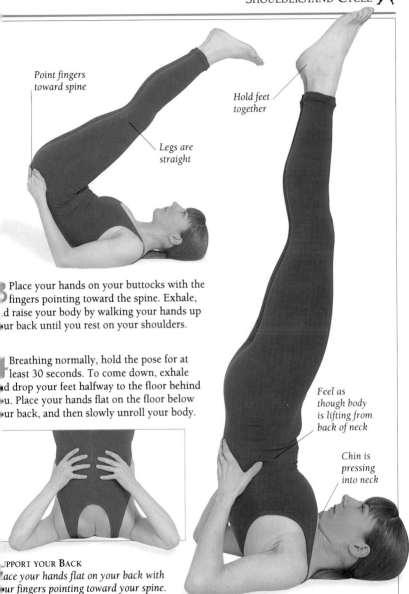

Point fingers toward spine

Legs are straight

Hold feet together

3 Place your hands on your buttocks with the fingers pointing toward the spine. Exhale, [an]d raise your body by walking your hands up [yo]ur back until you rest on your shoulders.

4 Breathing normally, hold the pose for at least 30 seconds. To come down, exhale [an]d drop your feet halfway to the floor behind [yo]u. Place your hands flat on the floor below [yo]ur back, and then slowly unroll your body.

Feel as though body is lifting from back of neck

Chin is pressing into neck

SUPPORT YOUR BACK
[Pl]ace your hands flat on your back with [yo]ur fingers pointing toward your spine.

31

50 PLOW

The Shoulderstand (see p.30) leads into the Plow, a position in which your feet touch the floor behind your head to create a powerful forward bending of the spine. The Plow increases overall flexibility, but it is particularly effective for relieving tension in the upper back and shoulders. As in the Shoulderstand, the chin rests on the neck and massages the thyroid.

Keep knees straight

1 Supporting your back, inhale deeply, and then exhale as you lower your legs.

2 When your feet touch the ground, lay your arms on the floor with the palms down. Hold for 30 seconds. Slowly roll out of the position.

Legs remain straight

Toes touch floor

EASING UP ▷
If, while practicing the Shoulderstand or the Plow, your legs start to tense up, bend your knees until they rest on your forehead. Support your back and breathe deeply. You will then be able to continue the cycle.

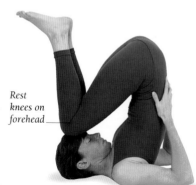

Rest knees on forehead

TAKING THE STRAIN
If you are unable to touch the floor with your toes in the Plow, be sure to keep supporting your back with your hands, to avoid straining your back muscles.

51 BRIDGE

The Bridge is a backward bend. Perform after the Plow to provide a complementary stretch of the thoracic and lumbar regions.

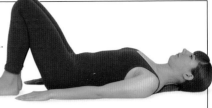

1 Starting from the Corpse Pose (*see p.24*), bend your knees and place your feet flat on the floor.

2 Place your hands on your back with your fingers pointing toward your spine. Lift your hips high. Hold this pose for 30 seconds.

Rest head and shoulders on the floor

Feet flat

52 FISH

From the Corpse Pose (*see p.24*), tuck your arms close in under your body. Tilt your head back until the crown rests on the floor. Inhale and arch your chest upward.

Hold for 30 seconds

Legs straight

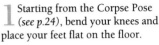

53 RELAX IN THE CORPSE POSE

After the Shoulderstand Cycle, relax in the Corpse Pose (*see p.24*) until your breathing has slowed and your heart rate has reached a resting level. Mentally check over the whole body to see if you can feel any areas of tension. Proceed with the yoga session when you feel ready.

33

FORWARD BENDS

54 PURPOSE OF THE FORWARD BENDS

Many of us spend most of our waking hours standing upright, and this can cause the spine to become compressed. Regular practice of the Forward Bends can help to keep the spine elastic, the joints mobile, the internal organs toned, and the nervous system invigorated.

55 HEAD TO KNEE

To achieve the Head to Knee pose, you must try to relax your body into the posture, rather than force yourself into it.

1 ▷ Start by sitting with your legs straight in front of you. Inhale and bring both arms up parallel to your ears. Stretch your spine. Lean forward from your hips, exhaling and keeping your spine and legs straight.

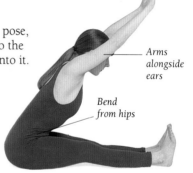

Arms alongside ears

Bend from hips

Keep spine as straight as possible

Avoid forcing down head

2 ▽ Draw your chest as close to your thighs as possible. Hold for 30 seconds, inhale, stretch up, and repeat the posture two to three times.

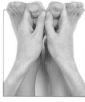

CORRECT HAND POSITION

Knees straight

Try to hold toes

56 ONE KNEE BENT

Many of us spend so much time sitting hunched over a desk or at the wheel of a car that our back muscles become shortened and weakened. This exercise stretches the back muscles, aiding proper alignment of the spine.

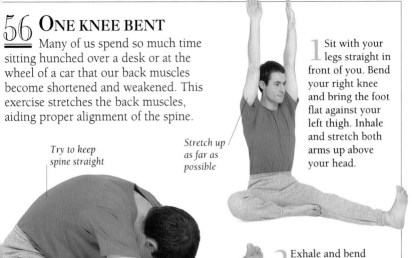

Stretch up as far as possible

Try to keep spine straight

1 Sit with your legs straight in front of you. Bend your right knee and bring the foot flat against your left thigh. Inhale and stretch both arms up above your head.

2 Exhale and bend forward over your straight leg. Grasp your toes. Hold for 30 seconds. Come up, inhaling, and repeat with the other leg.

57 LEGS APART

Sit with your legs spread wide apart. Inhale and raise your arms above your head. Exhale and stretch forward, trying to catch hold of the toes of both your feet. Bring your head down toward the floor.

Relax neck and allow head to hang down

Keep legs straight

Hold toes or ankles

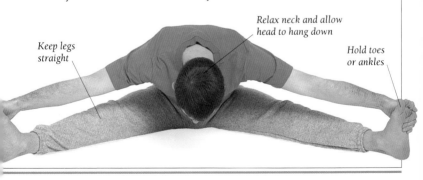

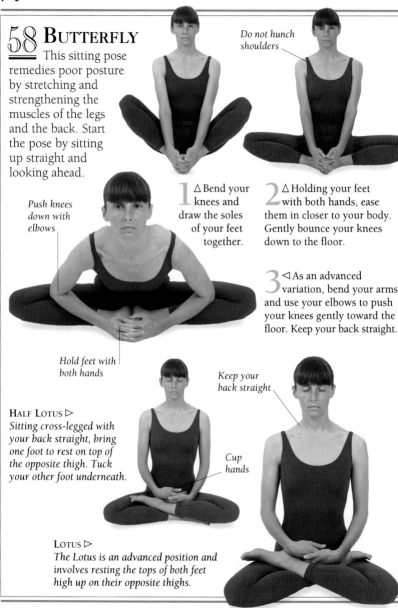

58 BUTTERFLY

This sitting pose remedies poor posture by stretching and strengthening the muscles of the legs and the back. Start the pose by sitting up straight and looking ahead.

Do not hunch shoulders

Push knees down with elbows

1 △ Bend your knees and draw the soles of your feet together.

2 △ Holding your feet with both hands, ease them in closer to your body. Gently bounce your knees down to the floor.

3 ◁ As an advanced variation, bend your arms and use your elbows to push your knees gently toward the floor. Keep your back straight.

Hold feet with both hands

HALF LOTUS ▷
Sitting cross-legged with your back straight, bring one foot to rest on top of the opposite thigh. Tuck your other foot underneath.

Keep your back straight

Cup hands

LOTUS ▷
The Lotus is an advanced position and involves resting the tops of both feet high up on their opposite thighs.

59 INCLINED PLANE

Immediately after a forward bend, counterpose the movement by stretching your spine back the other way in the Inclined Plane Position. This pose also serves to strengthen the shoulders, arms, and wrists.

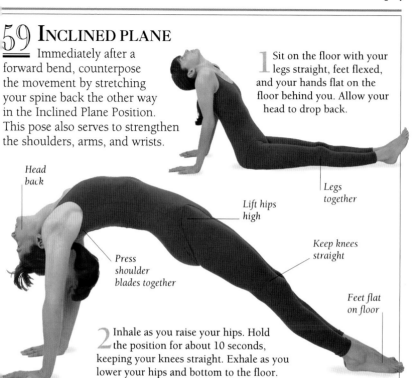

1 Sit on the floor with your legs straight, feet flexed, and your hands flat on the floor behind you. Allow your head to drop back.

Legs together

Head back

Lift hips high

Press shoulder blades together

Keep knees straight

Feet flat on floor

2 Inhale as you raise your hips. Hold the position for about 10 seconds, keeping your knees straight. Exhale as you lower your hips and bottom to the floor.

60 RELAX ON YOUR ABDOMEN

To relax between Backward Bends (*see p.38*), use this variation on the Corpse Pose (*see p.24*). Lie on your front and make your hands into a pillow on which to rest your head. Let your big toes touch, and allow your heels and ankles to fall gently out to either side. Breathe deeply.

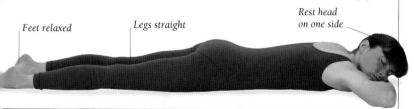

Feet relaxed

Legs straight

Rest head on one side

BACKWARD BENDS

61 COBRA

The Cobra is a face-down position in which you lift the upper body, curling up and back like the snake. By holding the posture, the deep and superficial muscles of both the back and abdominal region are toned and strengthened. It increases backward bending flexibility in your spinal column and relieves tension, particularly in the lower back region

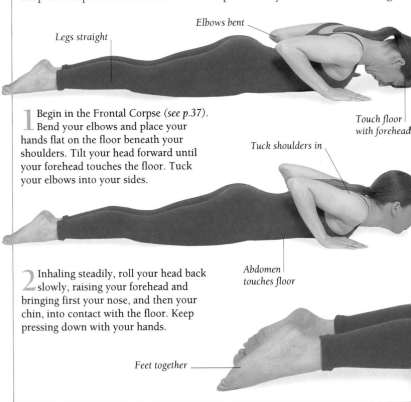

Legs straight

Elbows bent

Touch floor with forehead

1 Begin in the Frontal Corpse (*see p.37*). Bend your elbows and place your hands flat on the floor beneath your shoulders. Tilt your head forward until your forehead touches the floor. Tuck your elbows into your sides.

Tuck shoulders in

2 Inhaling steadily, roll your head back slowly, raising your forehead and bringing first your nose, and then your chin, into contact with the floor. Keep pressing down with your hands.

Abdomen touches floor

Feet together

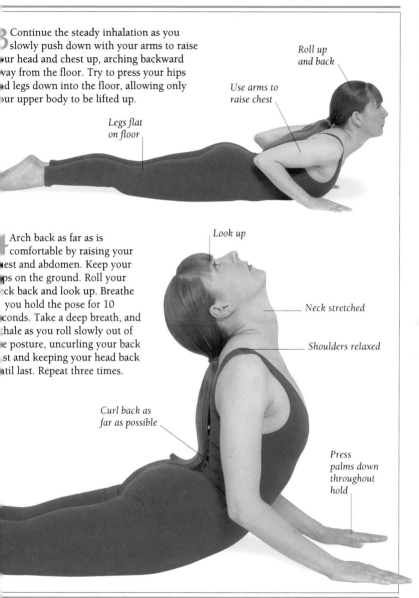

Continue the steady inhalation as you slowly push down with your arms to raise your head and chest up, arching backward away from the floor. Try to press your hips and legs down into the floor, allowing only your upper body to be lifted up.

Roll up and back

Use arms to raise chest

Legs flat on floor

Arch back as far as is comfortable by raising your chest and abdomen. Keep your hips on the ground. Roll your back back and look up. Breathe as you hold the pose for 10 seconds. Take a deep breath, and exhale as you roll slowly out of the posture, uncurling your back first and keeping your head back until last. Repeat three times.

Look up

Neck stretched

Shoulders relaxed

Curl back as far as possible

Press palms down throughout hold

62 LOCUST

This backward bending exercise increases the flexibility of the upper back and strengthens the lower back muscles. While holding the pose, the body weight is on the abdomen, and this stimulates and massages the internal organs.

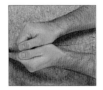

CLENCHED HANDS

CLASPED HANDS

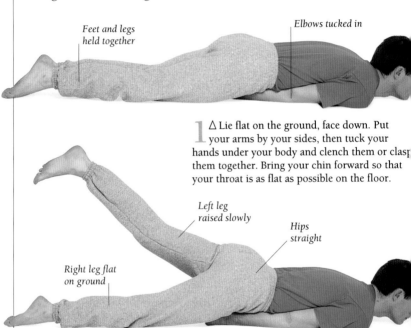

Feet and legs held together

Elbows tucked in

1 △ Lie flat on the ground, face down. Put your arms by your sides, then tuck your hands under your body and clench them or clasp them together. Bring your chin forward so that your throat is as flat as possible on the floor.

Left leg raised slowly

Hips straight

Right leg flat on ground

2 △ Inhale as you slowly raise your left leg, ensuring that your right leg remains flat on the floor. Keep both legs straight and make sure that your hips do not twist. Hold the lift for at least 10 seconds. Exhale as you gently lower the leg. Repeat the exercise with the right leg. Repeat two to three times for each leg.

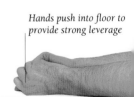

Hands push into floor to provide strong leverage

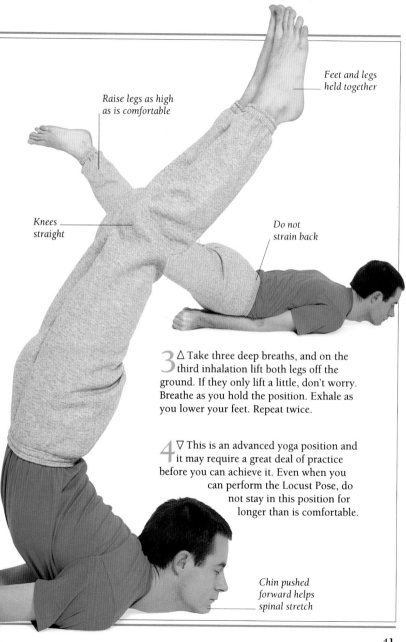

*Raise legs as high
as is comfortable*

*Feet and legs
held together*

*Knees
straight*

*Do not
strain back*

3 △ Take three deep breaths, and on the
third inhalation lift both legs off the
ground. If they only lift a little, don't worry.
Breathe as you hold the position. Exhale as
you lower your feet. Repeat twice.

4 ▽ This is an advanced yoga position and
it may require a great deal of practice
before you can achieve it. Even when you
can perform the Locust Pose, do
not stay in this position for
longer than is comfortable.

*Chin pushed
forward helps
spinal stretch*

63 Bow

The Bow works all parts of the back simultaneously, increasing strength and suppleness in the spine and the hips. While holding the pose, the arms are held taut, and this helps stretch the neck, leg, arm, and shoulder muscles. This backward bend combines the benefits of the Cobra (*see p.38*) and the Locust (*see p.40*).

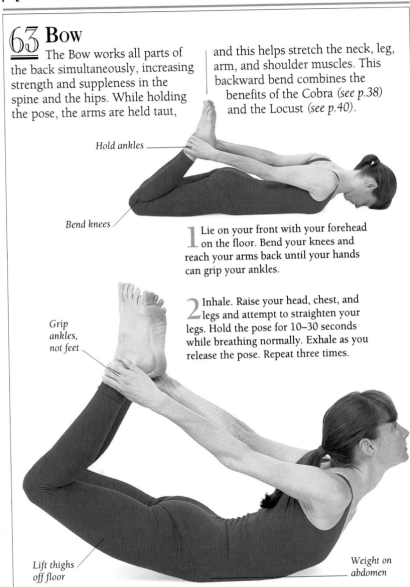

Hold ankles

Bend knees

1 Lie on your front with your forehead on the floor. Bend your knees and reach your arms back until your hands can grip your ankles.

2 Inhale. Raise your head, chest, and legs and attempt to straighten your legs. Hold the pose for 10–30 seconds while breathing normally. Exhale as you release the pose. Repeat three times.

Grip ankles, not feet

Lift thighs off floor

Weight on abdomen

64 CAMEL

The Camel enables you to exercise all of your back muscles and extend your spinal column, by bending your back fully. It is very useful for increasing spinal and hip flexibility.

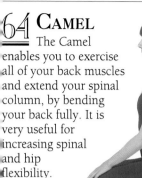

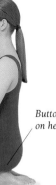

Buttocks on heels

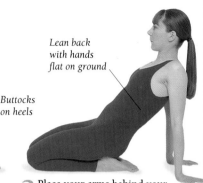

Lean back with hands flat on ground

1 Begin the posture by sitting on your heels. Keep your knees close together and your calves parallel with each other.

2 Place your arms behind your body with both palms flat on the floor. Lean back so that your weight rests on your hands.

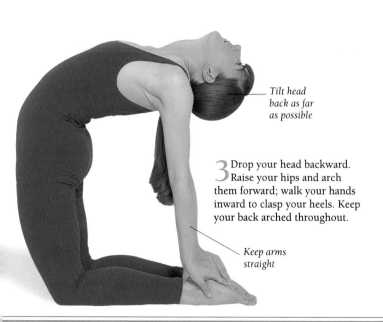

Tilt head back as far as possible

3 Drop your head backward. Raise your hips and arch them forward; walk your hands inward to clasp your heels. Keep your back arched throughout.

Keep arms straight

65 WHEEL

The Wheel may look difficult, but it is worth working at slowly and systematically, as it can bring great strength and flexibility to the spine and back muscles. Practice Steps 1 and 2 (Half Wheel) until the pose comes easily before proceeding to Steps 3 and 4 (Full Wheel).

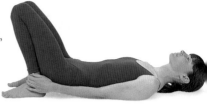

1 Lie on your back, bend your knees, and put your feet flat on the floor, near your buttocks. Hold your ankles.

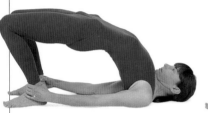

2 Grasp your ankles and push your hips up as far as possible. Keep your head, shoulders, and feet on the floor. Hold for 20 seconds. Lower your hips.

3 Put your hands flat on the floor behind your shoulders with the fingers pointing toward your shoulder blades.

4 Lift your hips, arching your entire spine and dropping your head back. Only your hands and feet remain planted on the floor. Aim to hold this posture for 30 seconds.

Try to straighten the knees as much as possible

Fingers point toward feet

Walk hands in toward feet

SPINAL TWISTS

66 INTRODUCTORY TWIST

After forward and backward bends (Tips 54–65), give the spine a lateral twist. This mobilizes the vertebrae and allows nourishment to reach the roots of the spinal nerves and the sympathetic nervous system. Relax in the Child's pose, kneeling with your forehead on the ground, before starting.

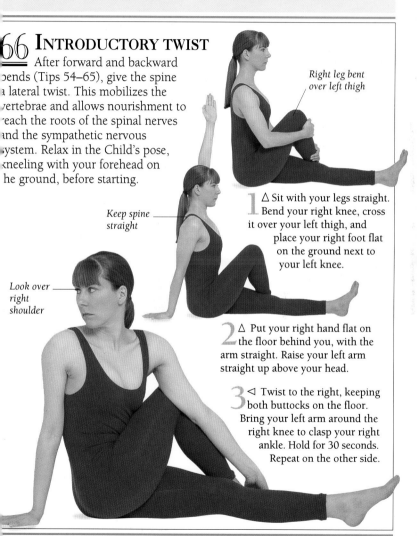

Right leg bent over left thigh

Keep spine straight

Look over right shoulder

1 △ Sit with your legs straight. Bend your right knee, cross it over your left thigh, and place your right foot flat on the ground next to your left knee.

2 △ Put your right hand flat on the floor behind you, with the arm straight. Raise your left arm straight up above your head.

3 ◁ Twist to the right, keeping both buttocks on the floor. Bring your left arm around the right knee to clasp your right ankle. Hold for 30 seconds. Repeat on the other side.

67 SPINAL TWIST

Side-to-side mobility is usually the first type of flexibility to be lost as our bodies become older. This posture stretches the spine, helping it to regain this mobility. As the vertebrae are mobilized, the roots of the spinal nerves and the nervous system are toned and provided with an increased blood supply. Work both sides of the body equally to gain the full benefit of the exercise.

Shoulders down and relaxed

1 ▷ In preparation for the Spinal Twist, sit on your heels. Knees and feet should be together, and the chest faces forward.

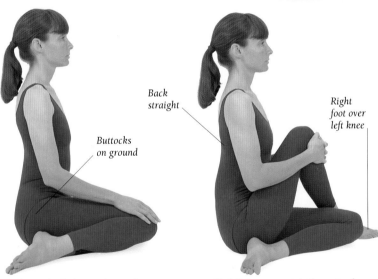

Back straight

Right foot over left knee

Buttocks on ground

2 △ Gently shift your buttocks down to the floor on the left side of your legs. Keep your back straight and centered over the buttocks.

3 △ Bring your right knee in close to your chest and gently lift it over your left leg; place the right foot flat on the floor by your left knee.

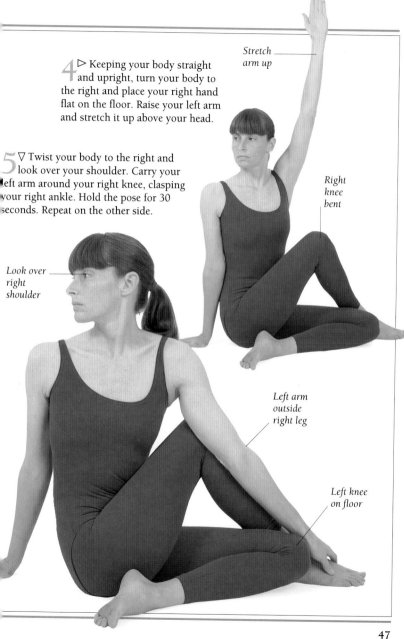

4 ▷ Keeping your body straight and upright, turn your body to the right and place your right hand flat on the floor. Raise your left arm and stretch it up above your head.

Stretch arm up

5 ▽ Twist your body to the right and look over your shoulder. Carry your left arm around your right knee, clasping your right ankle. Hold the pose for 30 seconds. Repeat on the other side.

Right knee bent

Look over right shoulder

Left arm outside right leg

Left knee on floor

BALANCING POSES

68 TREE

Balancing exercises demand strong concentration. The key to the Tree, and other balancing poses, is to focus on an external point, such as a mark on a wall, and to keep your attention on it. With practice, balancing will come easily.

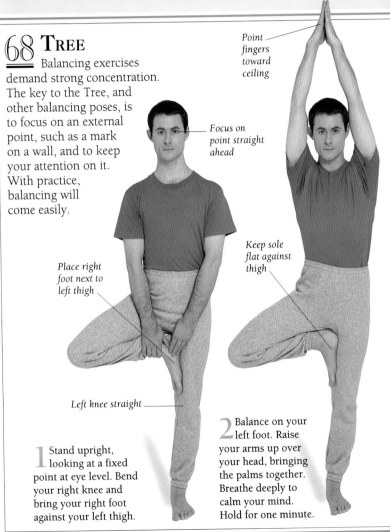

Point fingers toward ceiling

Focus on point straight ahead

Keep sole flat against thigh

Place right foot next to left thigh

Left knee straight

1 Stand upright, looking at a fixed point at eye level. Bend your right knee and bring your right foot against your left thigh.

2 Balance on your left foot. Raise your arms up over your head, bringing the palms together. Breathe deeply to calm your mind. Hold for one minute.

69 CROW

People who work at computers and typewriters often suffer from pain and stiffness in their wrists and forearms. The Crow can bring relief: it strengthens these areas. It also helps improve concentration and develop mental tranquillity.

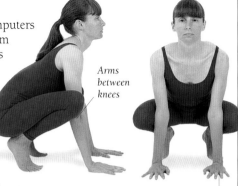

Arms between knees

Fingers stretched apart

1 △ Squat with feet and knees apart. Place your arms between your knees, with hands directly beneath your shoulders. Place your hands flat on the floor in front of you.

2 △ Bend the elbows and turn them outward. Rest your knees against your upper arms. Rock your body forward and feel the weight on your wrists.

Keep head up

Hands turned slightly inward

3 ▷ Slowly raise one foot, then the other. Balance on your hands for at least 10 seconds, gradually building up to one minute. To come out, lower your feet to the floor, and shake out your wrists. Repeat two or three times.

SECURITY CUSHION
Place a pillow on the floor in front of you if you are afraid of falling forward.

49

70 PEACOCK

This posture demands strength, flexibility, and concentration to be performed correctly. When the pose is held, your elbows press into the abdominal region, drawing fresh blood to the area and nourishing your internal organs.

Keep torso straight and relaxed

1 Start in the kneeling position, sitting on your heels with toes together and knees wide apart.

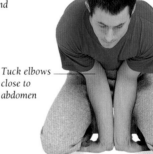

Tuck elbows close to abdomen

2 Place your arms between your legs, bringing your elbows and forearms together. Put your hands flat on the floor, with your wrists together and fingers pointing back toward your body.

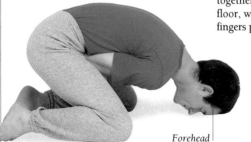

Forehead on floor

3 Bend your elbows into your abdomen, then allow the weight of your body to bear down on your elbows. Lower your forehead to the ground.

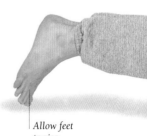

Allow feet to rise

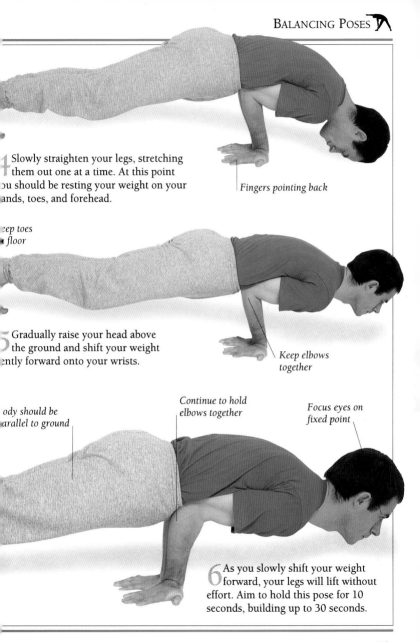

4 Slowly straighten your legs, stretching them out one at a time. At this point you should be resting your weight on your hands, toes, and forehead.

Fingers pointing back

Keep toes on floor

5 Gradually raise your head above the ground and shift your weight gently forward onto your wrists.

Keep elbows together

Continue to hold elbows together

Focus eyes on fixed point

Body should be parallel to ground

6 As you slowly shift your weight forward, your legs will lift without effort. Aim to hold this pose for 10 seconds, building up to 30 seconds.

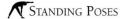
STANDING POSES

71 STANDING HANDS TO FEET

In this posture, you give a complete stretch to the back of the body. It is a simple but invigorating position, in which the joints are mobilized and the brain is supplied with an increased amount of blood. The pose also helps balance and correct inequalities in the body.

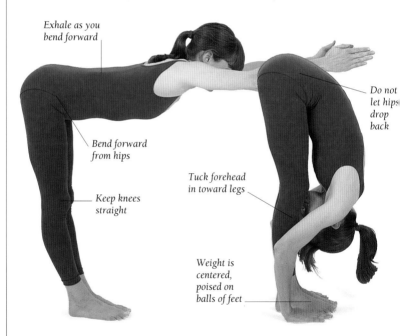

Exhale as you bend forward

Do not let hips drop back

Bend forward from hips

Tuck forehead in toward legs

Keep knees straight

Weight is centered, poised on balls of feet

1 Stand erect with your feet together. Inhale and stretch your arms above your head; hold them straight. Exhale and slowly start to bend forward, keeping your arms and legs straight.

2 Bend down. Catch hold of the backs of your legs and bring your head in as close to your legs as possible. Stretch your hips up. Breathe naturally. Hold for 30 seconds, increasing with experience.

72 TRIANGLE

The Triangle helps bring flexibility to the hips, shoulders, and legs. It stretches both sides of the body and gives a lateral stretch to the spine.

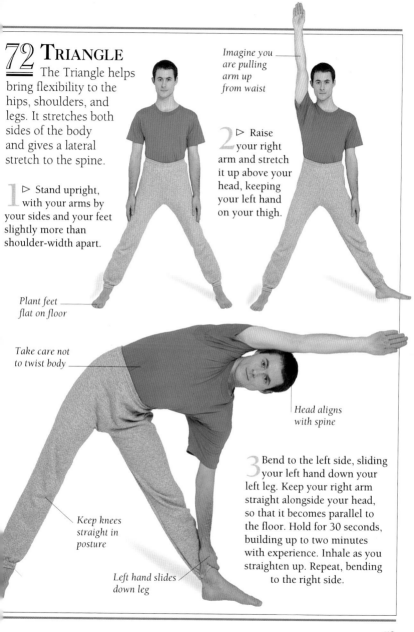

1 ▷ Stand upright, with your arms by your sides and your feet slightly more than shoulder-width apart.

Plant feet flat on floor

Imagine you are pulling arm up from waist

2 ▷ Raise your right arm and stretch it up above your head, keeping your left hand on your thigh.

Take care not to twist body

Head aligns with spine

Keep knees straight in posture

Left hand slides down leg

3 Bend to the left side, sliding your left hand down your left leg. Keep your right arm straight alongside your head, so that it becomes parallel to the floor. Hold for 30 seconds, building up to two minutes with experience. Inhale as you straighten up. Repeat, bending to the right side.

73 HEAD TO KNEE

Stand with your feet apart and clasp your hands behind your back. Turn to the left. Exhaling, lower your forehead to your left knee and lift your arms away from your back. Hold for at least 30 seconds. Inhale as you come up, returning to the starting position. Repeat, turning to the right.

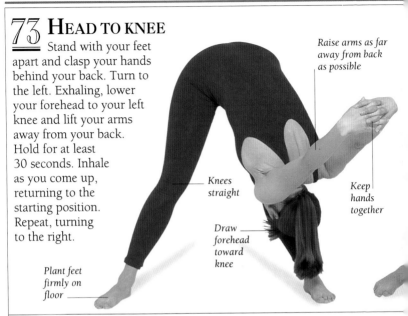

Raise arms as far away from back as possible

Knees straight

Keep hands together

Draw forehead toward knee

Plant feet firmly on floor

74 DEEP LUNGE

Stand with your feet wide apart and your hands clasped loosely behind your back. Turn your left foot out and bend your left knee until you are in a deep lunge. Lower your head to the floor inside your left foot and raise your hands as high as possible. Hold the pose for 30 seconds. Repeat for the right side.

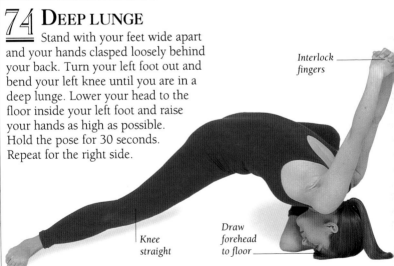

Interlock fingers

Knee straight

Draw forehead to floor

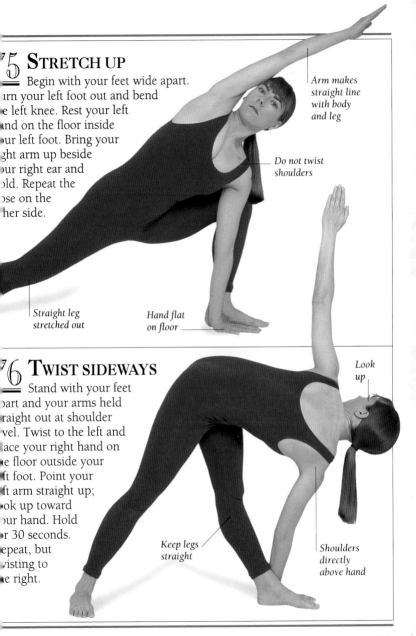

75 STRETCH UP

Begin with your feet wide apart.
Turn your left foot out and bend
the left knee. Rest your left
hand on the floor inside
your left foot. Bring your
right arm up beside
your right ear and
hold. Repeat the
pose on the
other side.

*Arm makes
straight line
with body
and leg*

*Do not twist
shoulders*

*Straight leg
stretched out*

*Hand flat
on floor*

76 TWIST SIDEWAYS

Stand with your feet
apart and your arms held
straight out at shoulder
level. Twist to the left and
place your right hand on
the floor outside your
left foot. Point your
left arm straight up;
look up toward
your hand. Hold
for 30 seconds.
Repeat, but
twisting to
the right.

*Look
up*

*Keep legs
straight*

*Shoulders
directly
above hand*

55

FINAL RELAXATION

77 WHY IS RELAXATION IMPORTANT?

Relaxing after the exercises can be the most important part of your yoga session. In addition to leaving you with a calm mind and relaxed muscles, the final relaxation allows your body to absorb the energy released by the asanas and to gain the full benefit from them.

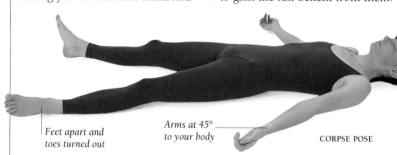

Feet apart and toes turned out

Arms at 45° to your body

CORPSE POSE

78 RELAX MENTALLY

Conscious relaxation is more of a mental exercise than a physical one. It involves sending mental messages to each part of your body, telling the muscles to tense up and then relax, while breathing gently and slowly. When all the muscles are relaxed, your mind, too, will feel calm. When you achieve a sense of inner peace, you can enter into this peace and become one with it.

79 FOR HOW LONG?

Final Relaxation is based on the Corpse Pose (see p.24), which should also be adopted before beginning your yoga session and between asanas. When you have completed a session, you should relax by resting in this pose for at least five minutes.

30 STEP-BY-STEP RELAXATION

Lie flat on your back in the Corpse Pose *(see p.24)*. Tense and relax the various muscles of your body following the steps shown. Then, without moving a muscle, mentally relax your body. Start by concentrating on the toes, and then move the relaxation up through the feet, legs, and all parts of the body, including the jaw, throat, tongue, and face. Finally relax your mind.

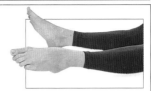

1 Raise each leg in turn 2 in (5 cm) from the floor. Tense the muscles and then "let go," allowing your foot to drop.

CLENCH FISTS   **SPREAD FINGERS**

2 Raise one arm, clench your fist, and allow your fingers to uncurl. Then spread your fingers wide and stretch them before allowing your hand to drop to the ground. Repeat the exercise with the other hand.

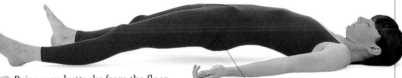

3 Raise your buttocks from the floor, tense the muscles, and then relax, allowing them to drop to the floor. Then raise your back and chest from the floor, tense, and relax.

Raise buttocks and tense them

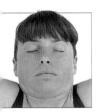 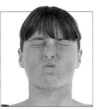 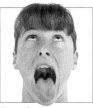 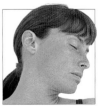

SHOULDER SHRUG
Pull your shoulders up, tense your neck muscles, and relax.

FACIAL MUSCLES
Tense the muscles of your face, mouth, and eyes; then relax.

FACE STRETCH
Open eyes and mouth wide, sticking your tongue out.

NECK ROLL
Turn your head from side to side twice, and return to the center.

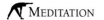

MEDITATION

81 WHY MEDITATE?

Meditation is beneficial for everyone, especially those with hectic, stressful lives. In meditation, the overactive mind is calmed and turned inward. This recharges the batteries, increases physical stamina and spiritual strength, and improves the powers of concentration. Regular meditation produces a clear mind and a sense of great inner peace.

82 WHAT IS MEDITATION?

To understand what true meditation is, consider a lake. When the surface of a lake is still you can see to the bottom clearly. When the surface is agitated by waves, this is impossible. The same is true of the mind. When it is still you may see and experience inner calm.

83 WHEN & WHERE TO MEDITATE

If meditating inside, choose a warm space, free from noisy distractions and clutter. If outside, choose a place where you feel safe and relaxed, and there is little extraneous activity to disturb you. You can practice meditation at any time of day or night, but try to get into a daily routine to make it easier to train your mind.

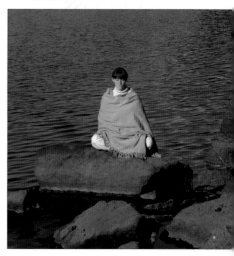

MEDITATING OUTSIDE ▷
Practicing in a place of natural beauty makes it easier to relax and prepare the body for the peaceful state of meditation.

84 COMFORTABLE CROSS-LEGGED POSITION

A comfortable sitting pose is very important if you are to meditate properly without distraction. Sit with your legs crossed and your spine erect. You should hold your shoulders straight, but relaxed. Children find this pose easy, but adults may need some assistance. Place a cushion under the buttocks to relieve any tension in the lower back. Advanced yoga students can sit in the Lotus Position (*see p.36*) during meditation.

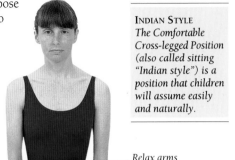

INDIAN STYLE
The Comfortable Cross-legged Position (also called sitting "Indian style") is a position that children will assume easily and naturally.

Relax arms

Legs should feel comfortable

85 HAND POSITIONS

The following positions are all suitable for meditation. Aim to hold your hands as comfortably as possible. This ensures that you remain relaxed while meditating. Resting your hands on your knees or in your lap also helps hold the spine straight and shoulders erect.

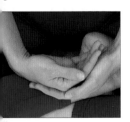

HANDS CUPPED
Place one hand on top of the other, palms upward, and lay them in your lap.

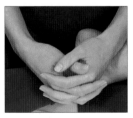

HANDS CLASPED
Clasp your hands gently by interlocking your fingers. Put your hands in your lap.

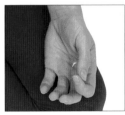

CHIN MUDRA
Use your thumb and first finger to form a circle. Rest your hands on your knees.

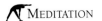

86 REGULATE YOUR BREATH

Breathing is a key element in meditation and concentration. Begin with 5 minutes of deep abdominal breathing, to provide your brain with plenty of oxygen. Then slow your breathing down, keeping it rhythmical, inhaling for 3 seconds and then exhaling for 3 seconds.

87 CONCENTRATION EXERCISE: TRATAK

To start this powerful yet easy concentration exercise, place a lit candle on a low table. Sit in a cross-legged position about 3 ft (1 m) away. Stare at the flame for about a minute, trying not to blink. Then close your eyes and visualize the flame at a point between your eyebrows. Try to focus your mind on this image for at least 1 minute. Repeat three to five times, increasing the visualizing time to 3 minutes.

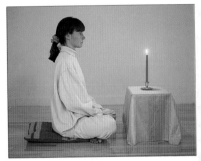

PRACTICING TRATAK

88 FOCUS ON A POINT

While meditating, you can focus on one of the body's chakras, or centers of spiritual energy, such as the Ajna Chakra, between the eyebrows, or the Anahata Chakra, near the heart. Repeat a personal mantra, or the mantra OM, each time you inhale and each time you exhale.

THE OM SYMBOL

89 IF YOUR MIND WANDERS...

At first you will find that your thoughts tend to jump around. Do not try to force your mind to be still; this will set additional brain waves in motion, hindering your meditation. Allow your mind to wander, and then gently command it to be calm. Focus your energy and attention inward by concentrating on an uplifting mental image.

ERADICATING BAD HABITS

00 STOP SMOKING

Yogic philosophy identifies two impure categories of foods – Rajasic (overstimulating) and Tamasic (stale or rotten). Tobacco is both. Giving up smoking eliminates toxins from the body and helps you achieve a calm mind and body.

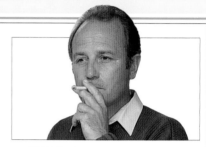

TOBACCO IS A POISONOUS STIMULANT

01 AVOID CAFFEINE

Caffeine is considered to be Rajasic, as it is a powerful stimulant. It causes the mind to be overactive and gives the body artificial energy. It can also disrupt your natural sleeping pattern, impairing your ability to relax. If you cut out tea and coffee from your diet, you will find that meditation becomes easier.

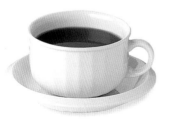

TEA AND COFFEE CONTAIN CAFFEINE

02 CUT OUT ALCOHOL

Alcohol contains fermented products, introducing toxins into the body, and it overexcites the mind. It is therefore both Tamasic and Rajasic. Eliminating alcohol from your diet will improve mental clarity and physical well-being.

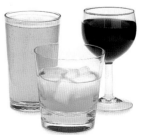

A YOGIC DIET EXCLUDES ALCOHOL

93 CHANGE YOUR DIET

In yogic philosophy, our diet affects far more than our physical well-being. Our vital energy, mental capabilities, and emotional health are all influenced by the food that we eat. The practice of meditation, postures, and breathing exercises is directed toward bringing the mind and the body into harmony. Eating the right foods is an important element in achieving this goal. Foods that are beneficial to us are said to Sattvic, or pure. Impure foods that can upset our physical, emotional, intellectual balance are identified as being in the categories Tamasic (stand or rotten) and Rajasic (stimulating). You should avoid these foods.

Avoid Tamasic Foods

Foods that are stale, tasteless, unripe, overripe, or putrified are Tamasic. They poison the body, sap our energy, and dull the intellect. Tamasic foods include meat and fish, mushrooms, and foods that have been frozen, preserved, canned, overcooked, or reheated. Foods that have been fermented, such as vinegar, are Tamasic, as are all drugs and alcohol. Eating too much is also considered to be Tamasic.

Avoid Rajasic Foods

Onions and garlic, tobacco, eggs, coffee, tea, hot peppers and other strong spices, and foods that are sour, acid, or bitter are all Rajasic. Chocolate, white sugar, white flour, and most prepared and convenience foods are also Rajasic to a lesser extent. All these substances excite the passions and overstimulate the mind, making it difficult to control. Eating too fast and eating too many combinations of food is also Rajasic.

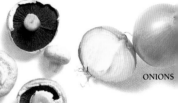

MUSHROOMS

CHILIES

GARLIC

SPICES

ONIONS

EGGS

FOODS THAT HINDER
As an aspiring student yoga, you need a diet will enable you to der the greatest benefit fr the yoga asanas and meditation exercises. All these food items a categorized as Tamas or Rajasic, and as suc they should be avoide a healthy body and m are to be kept in bala

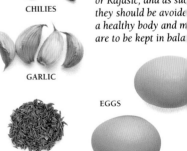

oose Sattvic Products

tvic foods form the ideal diet,
ng nourishing and easy to digest.
ey create new energy and a clear,
m mind, enabling us to use all our
ntal, physical, and spiritual talents.
tvic products include cereals, fresh
it and vegetables, natural fruit juices,
lk, butter, beans, honey, and pure water.

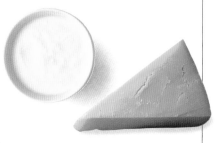

DAIRY PRODUCTS

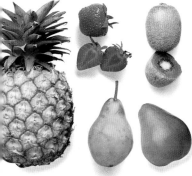

FRESH FRUIT

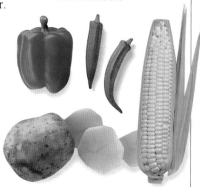

FRESH VEGETABLES

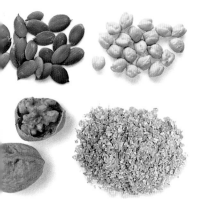

BEANS, NUTS, AND GRAINS

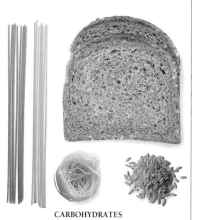

CARBOHYDRATES

SPECIAL PROGRAMS

94 IMPROVING YOUR CONCENTRATION

Our minds have a tendency to jump about constantly. This difficulty in concentrating cuts down on our efficiency. Work, study, and even recreational activities can be performed much better with full concentration. A student who can concentrate will achieve higher grades. A focused mind improves a golfer's game. Practicing simple yoga exercises will improve your concentration.

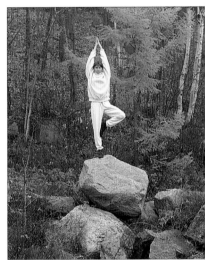

△ TREE
Positions that demand concentration and help improve it include the Tree (see p.48). Focus on a spot in front of you. Now mentally pull the spot in to rest between your eyebrows.

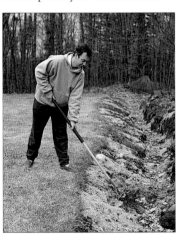

◁ CONCENTRATED RECREATION
The efficiency and the pleasure of an activity will be enhanced when approached with a calm and concentrated mind. Even a simple task in the garden can become an act of meditation.

95 STRESS MANAGEMENT

In addition to increasing your flexibility, the program of postures below will relieve stress by releasing tension that has built up in your body. Meditation exercises and breathing techniques can also be used as powerful tools for dealing with stress, as they both relax the body and calm the mind. Eating a vegetarian diet, not smoking, and avoiding stimulants all help to increase mental tranquillity.

COBRA

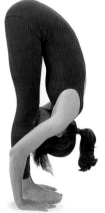

HEAD TO KNEES

Posture	For how long?
1. Headstand	1 minute
2. Shoulderstand	3 minutes
3. Plow	1–2 minutes
4. Bridge	½–1 minute
5. Fish	1½ minutes
6. Forward Bend	30 seconds x 3
7. Cobra	30 seconds x 3
8. Locust	30 seconds x 2
9. Bow	30 seconds x 3
10. Spinal Twist	½–1 minute each side
11. Head to Knees	1 minute
12. Triangle	30 seconds each side

96 OVERCOMING INSOMNIA

If you practice yoga regularly, you will find that your mind and body will gradually begin to develop more relaxed patterns of behavior. The yoga postures will reeducate the muscles and train them to relax.

Try to spend at least 30 minutes practicing each day. Regularity is of the utmost importance, and each session should begin with at least 5 minutes of relaxation and end with another 5 minutes. Be sure to relax between postures. If you have difficulty falling asleep at night, try repeating the Final Relaxation process (see p.56), mentally telling each part of your body in turn to tense up and then relax completely.

97 DURING PREGNANCY

The prenatal period, when your body and mind are engaged in the creation of a new life, can be a rare and valuable learning experience. Yoga can help you have an easier, healthier pregnancy and delivery. Practiced slowly and gently, the postures relax and strengthen the body, allowing you to adjust to many of the temporary physical changes. The breathing exercises can enable you to make the most of your breath.

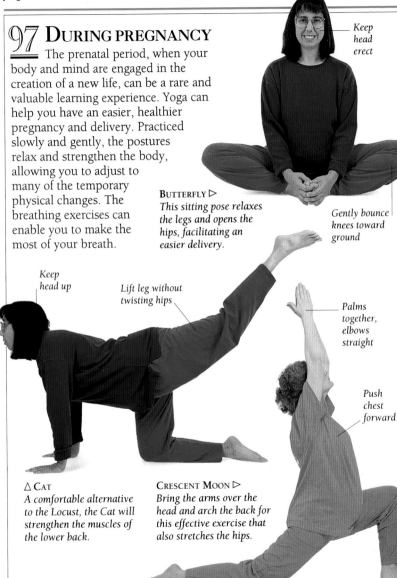

Keep head erect

BUTTERFLY ▷
This sitting pose relaxes the legs and opens the hips, facilitating an easier delivery.

Gently bounce knees toward ground

Keep head up

Lift leg without twisting hips

Palms together, elbows straight

Push chest forward

△ CAT
A comfortable alternative to the Locust, the Cat will strengthen the muscles of the lower back.

CRESCENT MOON ▷
Bring the arms over the head and arch the back for this effective exercise that also stretches the hips.

98 WHAT NOT TO DO WHEN PREGNANT

- Do not perform the Bow.
Do not attempt the Locust.
Shoulderstand and Plow should only be practiced if comfortable.
Do not perform the Cobra (or the seventh Sun Salutation position).

- Do not practice the Peacock.
- Do not perform the Headstand for the first time during pregnancy. If you are used to it, you can continue until it becomes uncomfortable (probably about the fourth month).

99 AFTER THE BABY IS BORN

After pregnancy you can assist your body in returning to its former physical condition as quickly as possible. You may begin (or return to) the postures and breathing exercises as soon as you like. Don't push yourself unnecessarily, but try to practice on a regular basis. Yoga may be performed at any time of the day (as long as you have not eaten for at least two hours), so you can easily arrange the timing to fit your new schedule.

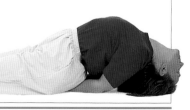

Clasp hands behind back

MODIFIED COBRA ▷
This has many of the benefits of the Cobra, but with no pressure on the abdomen.

SINGLE LEG LIFTS ▷
These will strengthen the lumbar region of the lower back and help your body recover quickly from the delivery.

FISH ▷
This pose will relieve tensions that may develop in the upper back and chest.

Keep feet together, but relaxed

100 YOGA AT ANY AGE

Yoga is suitable for everyone – young or old – and for all levels of fitness. Unlike many sporting activities, it is noncompetitive, so each person can work at his or her own pace. Since yoga is done very slowly, there is little risk of injury, providing it is done properly. Yoga helps people of all ages to maintain their good health and flexibility. It aids digestion, stimulates circulation, and lessens the effects of arthritis. Yoga helps teenagers keep their youthful flexibility throughout adult life, and its gentle movements are ideally suited to elderly people.

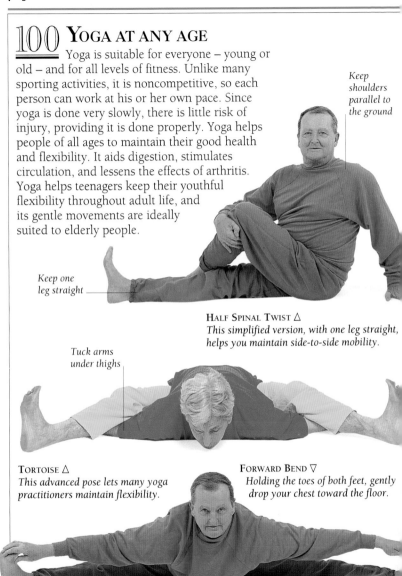

Keep shoulders parallel to the ground

Keep one leg straight

HALF SPINAL TWIST △
This simplified version, with one leg straight, helps you maintain side-to-side mobility.

Tuck arms under thighs

TORTOISE △
This advanced pose lets many yoga practitioners maintain flexibility.

FORWARD BEND ▽
Holding the toes of both feet, gently drop your chest toward the floor.

101 YOGA WITH CHILDREN

Yoga presents children with the opportunity to develop self-awareness, self-control, and better concentration. When children see yoga postures being practiced, their natural curiosity and love of mimicry often lead them to imitate.

Invite them to join you in your daily routine. You will probably find that they are very flexible but that they lack staying power. However, if the children are encouraged to practice on a regular basis, their mental control will improve greatly.

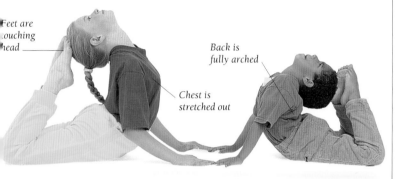

Feet are touching head

Back is fully arched

Chest is stretched out

FULL COBRA △
This pose demonstrates the natural agility of younger bodies. Through regular practice, yoga can help children to develop mental and physical self-control, as well as self-awareness.

FUN ▷
Yoga can be fun for both children and adults. It is a healthy and joyous event that you can experience together. Perhaps a regular time can be set aside for "family yoga" in the evenings or on weekends, when you are not rushed.

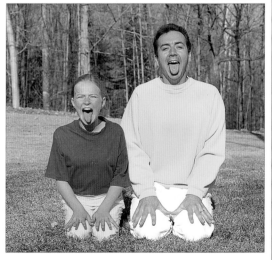

69

Index

ACKNOWLEDGMENTS

Dorling Kindersley would like to thank Rachel Leach,
Jenny Rayner, and Katie Bradshaw for picture research;
Ann Kay for proofreading; Hilary Bird for compiling the index;
Murdo Culver for design assistance; Swami Saradananda and
Ganapathi of the Sivananda Yoga Vedanta Centre, 51 Felsham Road,
London SW15 1AZ, for their help and advice throughout the project;
Chandra of the Sivananda Ashram Yoga Camp Headquarters in
Quebec, for his help on the photographic shoots; Amba, Shaun
Mould, Natalie Leucks, Adrienne Pratt, Satya Miller, Uma Miller,
Shambhavi, Annosha Reddy, Ishwara Proulx,
Chandra, and Fred Marks for modeling.

Photography
Andy Crawford and Jane Stockman,
with help from Paul Bricknell, Philip Dowall,
Alan Duns, Anthony Johnson, Dave King, David Murray,
Steven Oliver, Roger Phillips, and Clive Streeter.

Illustration
Simone End, Elaine Hewson, and Janos Marffy.

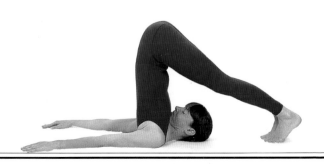